PRAISE FOR
JAMAICAN GREEN SMOOTHIES

"This is an excellent book for those looking to begin their health and wellness journey on a shoe string budget and improve even their skin tone. The recipes are simple and authentically Jamaican."
-- CAMEKA TAYLOR

"Excellent. Informative . Easy to read. Happy for the recipes."
-- JACQUELINE LYNCH-STEWART

"*Jamaican Green Smoothie* is a life-changer! My life has been and is being transformed. The smoothies have started a whole new lifestyle for me. The book and recipes are concise yet complete. A must read."
-- MICKEELA BROWN

"I have been interested in smoothies for a while but found it difficult and expensive to source ingredients in other books. This book is simple, easy to follow and best of all the recipes are fabulous and work well! After one week the difference is remarkable."
-- MARGARET CHRISTIAN

JAMAICAN GREEN SMOOTHIES

Jamaican Green Smoothies

The Essential Guide To Transforming Your Life, One Cup At A Time, With The Leafy Greens & Fruits In Your Backyard

By Didan Ashanta

Published by EarthStrong Publishing
12 Texas Avenue,
Portmore, Jamaica

For more information, see http://DidanAshanta.com/.

To the three young warriors,
who are growing up on Jamaican Green Smoothies,

Mwalimu

Bless'ed

Kinah

Acknowledgments

This process, from conception to final publication, has been very long and filled with many moments of celebration and frustration. I have been given much to be grateful for and have been supported and energised by many kind souls. This book could not have come into your possession without the concerted efforts of various persons and I am honoured to have been blessed to take this journey with them. I can only hope that this publication will bring them sufficient honour for their contributions and pray that it will be a constant reminder of my indebtedness to them.

First, I have to thank my husband, **Brad**, and daughter, **Mwalimu**, for drinking my various Jamaican Green Smoothie experiments and for tolerating my pre-occupation with this project and its various spinoffs. You both are my primary motivation for pursuing health and wellness, because I want us to enjoy each other for as long as possible, without the inconveniences, expenses and discomforts that come with disease.

I have to admit that this book would not have been conceptualized without the inspiration I received from a webinar hosted by **Dayna Wallace** and her partner, **Desriann Champagnie**, in May 2013. You, beautiful ladies, showed me how to embrace my passions and to share my knowledge and expertise with others. You took the time to interact with me personally and told me that my dreams were worth the effort. You are amazing women, who have dedicated your lives and work to enlightening and empowering your fellow Jamaicans, in ways that are yet to be matched. I hope *Jamaican Green Smoothies* will remind you both that your late nights and long days are worth it.

Half way through the writing of *Jamaican Green Smoothies*, my faithful laptop decided to announce its retirement. This was not just a threat to the completion of this book, but a major hindrance to my work as a freelance writer and online teacher. I'll forever be grateful to **Brad, Cameka, Eloretta, Jeannette, Mauricea, Shauna, Wilton and Yashi** for the gift of a brand new laptop for my birthday. It still means so much to me that, even during these difficult times, you made the sacrifices to help me fulfill my dream.

The most amazing support in this Jamaican Green Smoothie movement has come from all the **30-Day Jamaican Green Smoothie Challengers**. These are the men and women, living all across Jamaica and throughout the Jamaican diaspora, who have taken the plunge to drink a green smoothie, every day, for 30 days. We have gotten to know each other through the support group we've formed on Facebook and you are the most amazing group of people I have interacted with in a long time. Your daily posts of your Jamaican Green Smoothies and your gleeful announcements about weight loss, glowing skin, healthy hair, mental clarity, stamina, and the countless other benefits you've experienced were all the thanks I could ever need.

Heart-filled thanks to **Live Juice Bar, Real Farm Freshness and So Veggie** for providing the most fantastic deals, discounts and special offers to participants in the 30-Day Jamaican Green Smoothie Challenge. It is such an honour to have been able to partner with such generous and genuine people. I give your businesses my unreserved commendations because I know that you offer quality products and services and that you are passionately working to build Brand Jamaica. I am confident that we will see the health and wellness of our nation improve with every sale persons make with you.

Thank you to all the persons who attend my first **Live Webinar "The Jamaican Green Smoothie 101"** and to all the persons who have watched the recorded video that is posted for playback on my Youtube channel. Your support allowed me to expand my reach and to consider more ways of spreading the love for the green smoothie habit – Jamaican Style.

I'm still in awe and humbled by the opportunity to be featured on **Television Jamaica's Weekend Smile** morning programme, to talk about the 30-Day Jamaican Green Smoothie Challenge. It's not every day that your work gets noticed by the nation's number one media house, so I really want to thank the

Smile Jamaica producer, productions staff and hosts for giving us this platform. Special appreciation for my friends, **Suzanne and Cherie**, who gave up their chance to sleep in on Saturday morning so they could testify of the benefits of Jamaican Green Smoothies and demonstrate one of my recipes for the nation.

Thank you, **Daddy**, for taking those wonderful pictures of Jamaican leafy greens; and thank you, **Coronation Market vendors**, for allowing us to capture your vibrant produce. Special thanks to the **JGS Challengers** who freely shared their photos as with me in our vibrant support group. Thank you, **Jamellia**, for introducing me to Microsoft Word Online during those final weeks when I needed to proofread, edit and format on-the-go.

I am eternally grateful to my friend of many years and a dedicated professional in the field of Nutrition and Dietetics, **Yanique Rodgers**. I am truly honoured to have received your expert review of this book and completely humbled by your decision to give it your full endorsement by writing the foreward. Thanks a million, sis!

I can't close out this 'award ceremony' without paying honour to my Celebrity friends and colleagues who paid me the privilege of publishing their favourite Jamaican Green Smoothie recipes for your blending pleasure: **Bena, Brian, Camaley, Cherie, Cheryl, Clifton, Dayna, Jacqui, Jo-Ann, Kamaaleo, Mamayashi, Michael, Monique, Sabriya, and Stacey**. It gives me great joy to expose the Jamaican public to your love for green smoothies, so they can see that it abounds in all sectors of our society. Please be sure to try each of these lovely recipes – enough to keep you blending for 2 weeks, without any repeats. Just be warned: blending green smoothies is contagious!

-- Didan Ashanta

Table of Contents

Preface

The first time I encountered a green beverage was in January 2010, when I curiously purchased a bottle of Callaloo Juice from a supermarket in Spanish Town. After excitedly gulping down and draining the pint, I was extremely impressed and quickly convinced that green beverages could and were supposed to taste good. In the years that followed, I took note of friends and acquaintances who were extracting green juices and blending green smoothies, and I became particularly interested in learning to make my own green beverages because of my love for plant-based foods, health and wellness. It wasn't long before I noticed that all the social media platforms and wellness blogs were full of recipes and it seemed like every day someone was posting pictures of green smoothies. Even a friend started posting about her weight loss journey, using green smoothies. But, as I began to look around the internet at various green smoothie recipes, guides and ideas, I grew a bit indifferent because they all listed leafy green vegetables and fruits that I had never seen nor heard of in Jamaica; and if they had even been imported to some of the major supermarkets, they were quite expensive, e.g. kale, spinach, swiss chard, collards, mustard greens, peaches, raspberries, blueberries, strawberries, kiwi, etc. At around the same time, Live Juice Bar came on the scene, serving up green smoothies made from locally-grown Jamaican leafy greens and fruits; and I figured, I could try to make up my own green smoothie recipes.

One of my first blog posts on DidanAshanta.com just happened to be about my experimenting with Jamaican leafy greens and fruits to make green smoothies. The blends I had been making were quite delicious and I decided to share my experience with others. I realised that I never needed to complicate the green smoothie habit with a shopping list of foreign ingredients and superfoods, because a green smoothie was just a blend of leafy greens and fruits. So, I compiled and posted a quick list of the Jamaican leafy greens, fruits, liquids and extras that I was accustomed to having at home and encouraged my readers to check their refrigerators, backyards, farmers' markets and green grocers for their own green smoothie stash. Soon, I was blogging about taking a 30-Day Green Smoothie Challenge and even sharing tips & guidelines with other Jamaicans who had joined me on the journey of exploring the wonders of the Jamaican Green Smoothie. But, the lack of green smoothie recipes using Jamaican leafy greens and fruits, led to a few unpleasant blends and hilarious experiments for some of my readers. Fortunately, I love developing recipes and started writing down my favourite Jamaican Green Smoothie blends.

By the end of the July 30-Day Jamaican Green Smoothie Challenge, we couldn't help but realise that a green smoothie habit is a very efficient way to encourage healthy eating habits, and an excellent solution for those who struggle with food addictions. In the process, I learned a lot about the what, why and how of green smoothies and knew I had to find a way to share the wonders of this green goodness with others. But, there was no Green Smoothie guidebook nor recipe book for me to recommend to my readers, friends or associates that referenced the ingredients we eat and grow here in Jamaica. So, I decided that it was my job to fix that problem and bring, not just recipes but, the essential knowledge of green smoothies to my fellow Jamaicans.

-- Didan Ashanta

Foreword

As a Nutrition Science Professional, I have seen firsthand what scant regard persons pay to liquid nutrition. Many Jamaicans hold firmly to the belief that in order for a meal to be nutritious, it must comprise of "cooked" foods. Certainly, this belief leaves little room for the functionality and nutritional content of beverages. The few exceptions to this belief include: "roots" beverages made from herbs such as "Strong Back and "Horny Goat Weed"; along with Granny's favourite "bush" teas, such as the back-to-school staple, Cerasee Tea. But how many of us stop to consider the nutritive value of beverages? It is easier to drink than it is to eat, and this fuels the tendency of persons being more mindful of what they eat, than what they drink. Additionally, beverages are usually sweetened and Jamaicans have an insatiable sweet tooth, as evidenced by our love for mangoes - particularly the very sweet East Indian variety. This is why I am so excited about the concept of the Jamaican Green Smoothie, which encourages people to drink their fruits and vegetables! Wouldn't it be good to get all the nutritious goodness of vegetables in a tasty liquid form? I suspect this was the concept my father had in mind when he first decided to blend vegetables, like callaloo, lettuce and cucumbers together with water. He would then drink this concoction, straight from the blender without straining, before offering me a cup: to which, I would *mek up mi face* (make a face). Although, I knew Didan Ashanta at that time, unfortunately, she had not yet published this book, or even come up with her recipes for Jamaican Green Smoothies. Oh! How I look back on those days and wish my father had even added some June plums to the mix - just to sweeten it a bit.

Green smoothies allow for the natural goodness of vegetables and fruits to be incorporated into a beverage; and since there is no straining (leaving the fiber intact), they allow for the synergistic benefits that come with consuming whole foods. With all the wholesome, tasty nutrition found in green smoothies, persons may be tempted to overindulge in the hopes of curing whatever may ail them. But, as Granny used to say, *"Too much callaloo mek peppapot stew bitta"* or *"Too much a one ting, good fi nuttin."* So, we know that too much of a good thing can be bad; and that's why I especially appreciate that Didan included a chapter on the potential hazards of consuming green smoothies, and how to avoid same. When Didan first asked me to review this book, I was impressed with the depth of work and research she obviously put into writing it. No doubt, her experience in the food industry was of great help, particularly in the development of the recipes. The preface makes it clear that she saw a need, and instead of lamenting the dearth of green smoothie recipes, that utilise locally available ingredients, she took steps to meet that need. This, she did while further complementing the wellness-oriented lifestyle she is known for. She has even gone further, by engaging Jamaicans to develop the green smoothie habit, by inviting us to take on the 30 day Jamaican green smoothie challenge.

Had our parents recognised the value of liquid nutrition, perhaps some of us could have escaped being forced to eat a cooked meal of callaloo and pakchoy for breakfast. Instead of forcing our children to do the same, why not start a new tradition of having a green smoothie with, or for breakfast - or any other meal? It will certainly be much easier to lead by example with this new tradition. As our families build the tradition of drinking green smoothies, we will develop tasty, healthy, sustainable habits in ourselves and our children. I'm sure even Granny would approve.

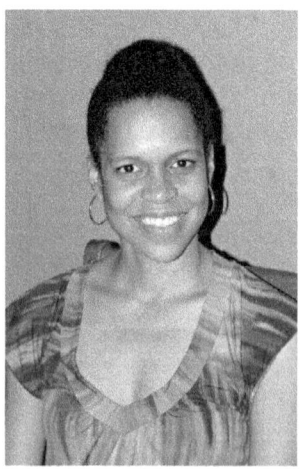

Yanique Rodgers
Food and Nutrition Scientist

Introduction

For quite some time, Jamaica's Health Minister, Hon. Dr. Fenton Ferguson, has been commenting on the epidemic of non-communicable diseases (NCD) in the nation, and has been urging us to take on healthier lifestyles to combat this problem. Lifestyle-related chronic diseases like cancer, diabetes, hypertension and heart disease are responsible for 70% of the loved ones and associates that we have to bury every year![1] In addition to telling us to reduce our consumption of alcoholic beverages, quit smoking, and increase our physical activity, medical professionals and nutritional experts have been reciting, like a scratched record, the mantra of 'eat more fruits and vegetables'. At the same time, the influence of the health and wellness industry has been expanding and in many social circles, eating healthy has become trendy. But, for most of us, adopting a healthier lifestyle is a major challenge. We want to improve our quality of life and avoid chronic lifestyle diseases, but we find it hard to eat a balanced diet because we are too busy to make most of our meals at home; the 'healthy' foods we have come across are not tasty; and even if we find great tasting food that is good for us, it tends to be much more expensive than we think we can afford. So, we are left to continue living with digestive problems, skin disorders, and reproductive health issues, and constantly battling problems with our weight, energy levels, and mental clarity, among other illnesses. The reality is that most of the diets we've seen being promoted as healthier, are filled with dietary restrictions and require too much effort to give them the time of day. After all, a healthier lifestyle should be simpler, shouldn't it?

A daily green smoothie is a habit that has been proven to transform lives by restoring one's health and improving one's sense of well-being. This practice of blending dark, green leafy vegetables with fruits into yummy emulsions has been trending across North America and the UK, with a wide range of

---

[1] The Editor. "Jamaica Faces Non-Communicable Disease Epidemic - Ferguson." *The Jamaica Gleaner* 13 Mar. 2014: News. The Gleaner. Web. 5 May 2014.

documented health benefits and prominent advocates. However, of the thousands of recipes that fill the internet and hundreds of green smoothie recipe books, very few could be replicated by Jamaicans without us investing in some costly and imported ingredients. So, if you browse the internet, you will find a trickling of Jamaicans who testify to adopting a green smoothie habit, or at least to developing an appreciation of the beverage. That is why this healthful and worthwhile blending habit has not caught on so easily in Jamaica; because most of us have no idea where to find the ingredients in most of these recipes; and when we do find them, it isn't the most affordable habit to pick up. But, after looking at the research, I still wanted to add these healthy beverages to my diet; so I took another look at the green smoothie and decided that since we Jamaicans regularly enjoy our own bunches of dark, green leafy vegetables, sautéed for breakfast, we should be able to throw them into the blender, as well. This is why I have explored Jamaican farms, backyard gardens, and produce markets to uncover the locally-grown, widely-available and nutrient-dense ingredients we have in Jamaica, that can be blended into green smoothies, at little or no cost to us to all of us. Then, after experimenting with a few of our green leaves, and finding yummy cup after yummy cup, I decided to share these delicious Jamaican Green Smoothies with you!

Jamaican Green Smoothies: The Essential Guide to Transforming Your Life, One Cup At a Time, With the Leafy Greens & Fruits in Your Backyard will help you to:
- Learn what green smoothies are and how to make them.
- Discover the benefits of a green smoothie habit and be equipped to avoid the potential hazards.
- Explore over 30 recipes - **a different Jamaican Green Smoothie for each day of the month** - including recipes for a Daily Habit, Weekend Treats, a One-Week Detox, and a Meal Replacement Weight Loss Plan.

The recipes that you will find in *Jamaican Green Smoothies* are one of a kind because they show you how to make green Smoothies that:
- Use affordable or free, locally-grown ingredients (leafy greens, fruits, liquids, herbs, spices).
- Take 5 minutes or less of your day to make.

- Are delicious, yet satisfy your daily requirement for fruit and vegetable intake.
- Will certainly balance your health and improve your lifestyle, without placing any dietary restrictions on you.

Jamaican Green Smoothies also includes **15 BONUS Celebrity Gourmet Recipes**! This additional features some favourite Jamaican Green Smoothie blends that were created by some prominent, yet regular Jamaican men and women, who have been enjoying the Green Smoothie habit for a long time and continue to reap the benefits.

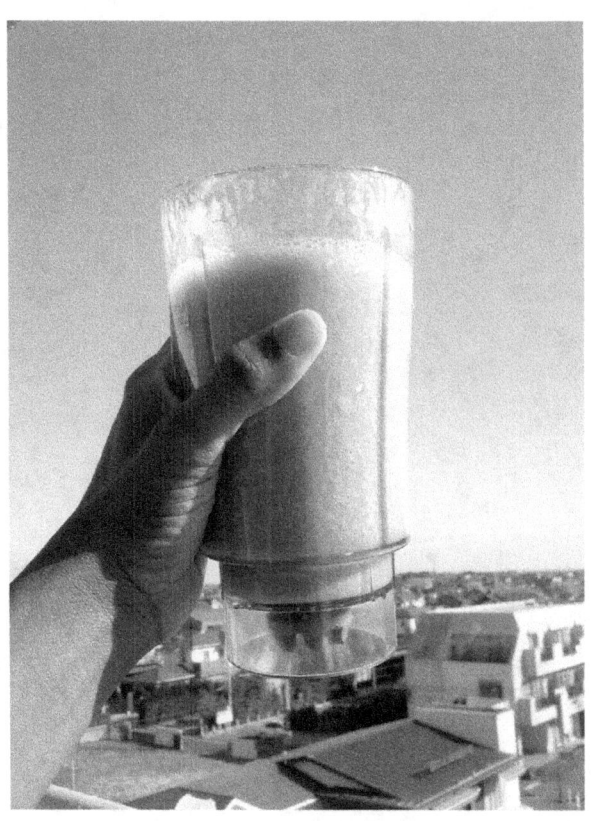

1.

Meet The Green Smoothie

What is a Green Smoothie?

A green smoothie is a cold beverage that is made by blending uncooked green, leafy vegetables (like Spinach, Kale, and Callaloo) with fruits (like Ripe Banana, Mango, and Pineapple) and liquids (like Water, Almond Milk and Grapefruit Juice). It is most often green in colour, but can be a variety of other colours depending on the quantity and type of green leaves used, as well as the quantity and colour/pigment of the fruit used. For example, enough Mango or Pawpaw may produce a golden orange smoothie, while loads of Blueberries or Otaheite Apple may give you a purple smoothie. The best green smoothies are thick, creamy and filling, so much so that they may be used as meal replacements; and if the fruit-to-leaf ratio is right, they will taste just like regular fruit-only smoothies.

The History of the Green Smoothie

Life in old time Jamaica saw us enjoying a Sky Juice (shaved ice and water topped with brightly coloured, fruit-flavoured syrup in a bag with a straw) on a sweltering, hot day. But, as our consciousness of health and wellness increased, we changed old habits and today, we've grown accustomed to consuming Fruit Slush, instead - those thick, sweet blends of fruit, fruit juice or fruit-flavoured syrup and ice. This refreshing blend is popularly known as a smoothie in the United States of America; and smoothies are an easy and delicious way to incorporate more fruit in our diets. Many persons blend them up every morning - even as a breakfast replacement. But, the wellness industry still encouraged us to develop even healthier habits, by increasing our consumption of dark green, leafy vegetables. So, very quickly green juices became popular and soon after, the green smoothie was born and it has been trending since.

Dr. Ann Wigmore, known as "the mother of living foods", was a pioneer in the raw food movement and she developed wonderful nut milks and seed cheeses that are still popular today. This Lithuanian Holistic Medical Practitioner also introduced the world to the wonders of wheatgrass, and according to the Ann Wigmore Natural Health Institute, Inc., she promoted fresh wheatgrass juice as "an effective healer because it contains chlorophyll, all minerals known to man, and vitamins A, B-complex, C, E, and K."[2] Dr. Wigmore also developed the Hippocrates diet, and advocated juicing fruits and vegetables as a way to obtain optimal nourishment. But, in her later years in life, she wrote:

> "*You may have noticed that I no longer advocate juicing, except for wheatgrass and watermelon juice. Juices such as green drinks can be too cleansing for most people's bodies which have become extremely toxic from environmental and dietary abuse. Blending helps the body to clean itself and thus it restores health much quicker than just eating the foods as salads, yet it does not overtax the system with the rapid cleansing action of juices. Eating nutritionally balanced food in a blended form is a big help to the immune system and thus even seems to overcome "incurable" health problems.*"[3]

This little bit of history is the reason many green smoothie experts recognise Dr. Wigmore as the inventor of the blending concept behind the green smoothie. However, it was Victoria Boutenko whose pioneering made the 'green smoothie' famous. In 2004, while researching the perfect diet for humans, Victoria tried to liquefy her green leaves, but she didn't like the taste. It was only after observing a chimpanzee wrap some fruit in the green leaves before eating them, that she thought of adding fruit to her blended

---

[2] "Living Foods Lifestyle," Ann Wigmore Natural Health Institute, Inc., accessed May 4, 2014, http://www.annwigmore.org/living_foods.html.
[3] Ann Wigmore, *Rebuild Your Health: With High Energy Enzyme Nourishment* (New Mexico: Ann Wigmore Foundation, 1991).

green leaves. Her book, *Green for Life: The Updated Classic on Green Smoothie Nutrition*, and the follow-up, *Green Smoothie Revolution: The Radical Leap Toward Natural Health*, are excellent reference tools for anyone wanting to dive deep into the world of green smoothies.

It seems that while health-food enthusiasts were busy chugging down bitter-tasting green juices and the rest of us were experimenting with small salads, the first green smoothie was being blended up by Victoria Boutenko, just by adding ripe bananas to her blender full of liquefied green leaves. This minor discovery has resulted in a major revolution and I have also come to agree that green smoothies are the perfect dietary habit for everyone and anyone who hopes to adopt and maintain a healthy diet without making sacrifices to the taste of their food or to their lifestyle.

Tools For Making a Green Smoothie

A green smoothie is so simple to make that you could make it with only one tool - *a blender*! That's it. Don't believe me? Let's break it down. You start by throwing some leaves into your blender and breaking up pieces of fruit then adding some water and blending. *Voila*! You've blended up a green smoothie with only a blender. But, there are a couple other kitchen utensils that we may use, along with a blender, to smooth out the process some more:

- **Kitchen Knife** - the blade must be sharp enough to slice through the ingredients easily.

- **Cutting Board** - to have a sturdy, sanitary surface for cutting up the ingredients.

- **Citrus Juicer** - to easily add freshly, squeezed citrus juices to a green smoothie.

- **Measuring Cup** - for measuring liquids like coconut milk and solids like fruits and leaves.

- **Measuring Spoons** - for measuring extras like ginger, flaxseed or honey.

- **Nutmeg Grater** - for shaving extras like cinnamon, nutmeg, citrus rinds, or dried coconut.

- **Spatula** - to scrape the sides of the blender jar when pouring out the smoothie.

It is very possible to start the green smoothie habit and continue it without most of these items, but they will prove helpful to a novice trying to get their portions right or a culinarian trying to develop new green smoothie recipes. Either way, these fruity-leafy emulsions will not happen without a blender. So, it's important to understand the different types of blenders so you can decide which one is right for you (if you don't already have one collecting dust in some corner or cupboard in your home).

The Blender

Yes, the most important gadget - and the only required tool - for your kitchen, workspace, or any other location you plan to make green smoothies in, is a blender. It is the blender's rotating metal blade(s) which turns edible green leaves and chunks of fruit into the smooth, creamy beverage you will love to make day-after-day. If you already have access to a blender, there is no need to get another. But, if you don't already have a blender, a visit to your local dealer in kitchen appliances will expose you to a wide variety of blenders. Just remember that, selecting one shouldn't be a complicated process. As you check around, you might find the following options available:

A.   **Countertop Blender** - This is the most common blender that you'll find, in most kitchens. The *Standard/Full-Sized* models may be designed with a single switch, while others come with various options like grind, mash, purée, liquefy and whip. The *High-Speed* models are so powerful that they can crush ice or pulverise chunks of concrete and wood! Okay... So, we don't need to do any construction work with our blenders, but these high-performance, heavy-duty devices eliminate the need for cutting up the ingredients or worrying about the smoothness of the beverage when blended.

B. **Personal Blender** - This is a mini-sized, single-serving blender that is light-weight, takes up little space and can still do the job pretty well. It's mainly designed for you to make single serving portions of your favourite beverage - and have it on the go! Many models even come with screw-on cup rims that allow for comfortable sipping straight from the blending container. These blenders very often require you to cut your ingredients into much smaller sizes for quick and efficient blending, but some are sturdy enough to crush ice cubes.

C. **Hand Blender** - This the immersion/stick blender that allows you to blend your ingredients in any container of your choice. For example, soup cans, mixing bowls or glass jars. They are not the most popular for blending beverages, but they work none-the-less.

Most green smoothie advocates and experts will recommend that you get an expensive, high powered blender, while tossing brand-names like Vitamix, Blendtec and Breville at you. But, these expensive, high-powered blenders are not a requirement for you to blend up your first green smoothie, and not having one will not prevent you for forming a daily green smoothie habit. The most important thing to consider is that you are blending away so that you can fill up on the nutrient-richness of the various dark, green leafy vegetables. So, I encourage you to use whatever you have or buy whatever you can afford!

Living healthy does not mean you need to be wealthy

- it means that you need to be wise.

Juice vs Smoothie: Which is Better?

Most people are familiar with fruit juices, vegetable juices and green juices, but a juice is very different from a smoothie. To make juice, for example carrot juice, some persons may grate the carrot then use a sieve or muslin cloth to squeeze out the liquids. However, most persons just blend the carrot then strain away the pulp or trash, while other persons use a juice extractor to get the job done. In all three (3) cases, the fibrous matter from the fruit, vegetable or green leaves is separated from the liquids and frequently dumped. But when making smoothies, the ingredients are not strained, sieved nor the fibre extracted in any way. Instead, the ingredients are all blended together until they make a smooth and creamy drink - *no waste to discard and no time lost cleaning up.*

In her article, "To Juice or Blend?" Kristine Miles, author of "The Green Smoothie Bible" and writer at greensmoothiecommunity.com, explains the difference between a juice and a smoothie this way, "Juices do not contain fibre, so their nutrients are absorbed very quickly, high in the digestive tract... Smoothies are essentially juices with blended fibre - and it is the presence of fibre in smoothies that proponents of the drinks point to as their main virtue."[4] She went on to further expand the point by showing how a commonly eaten fruit moves through the digestive system depending on the form in which it is consumed:

> "Let's look at an orange consumed three ways: juiced, blended, and eaten. Orange juice requires no chewing and little or no energy beyond the stomach, and all of the sugars, vitamins, minerals, and antioxidants are available immediately and absorbed quickly into the bloodstream. A blended orange requires no chewing and minimal energy in the stomach and intestines, since the fibre has already been broken down into very small and functional pieces. The same nutrients as in the juice

---

[4] Kristine Miles, "To Juice or Blend?" The Green Smoothie Community, February 20, 2012.
http://greensmoothiecommunity.com/2012/02/20/to-juice-or-blend-2/.

are absorbed more slowly, and the sugars are released more slowly into the bloodstream because of the presence of soluble fibre. By comparison, eating an orange requires breaking down all of the constituents into smaller pieces, starting with chewing, then churning in the stomach, and further liquefying in the intestines so the fibre is small enough to do its job and the nutrients and sugars are small enough to be absorbed."[5]

You may read the rest of her article for more details on the benefits that one gains from both juices and smoothies. But, Kristine isn't the first or only person to discuss juicing versus blending. Dr. Wigmore wrote of juicing:

"Juices do not contain fiber. Separating the fiber and other elements from the juice results in a food that is not as balanced as Nature would have it. Nature provides us with complete foods in a perfectly complete package."[6]

While Victoria Boutenko wrote:

"One of the main advantages of juice is that it requires next to no digestion and can be absorbed and assimilated immediately into the bloodstream, allowing the digestive system to rest. This important quality of juice allows it to be used by people who suffer from severe nutritional deficiencies or have highly irritable digestive system. People with these conditions often cannot tolerate any fiber at all, and juice may provide invaluable nourishment for them. Later, when their health will improve, these people can switch to drinking smoothies...
I agree with Dr. Doug Graham that juices are a fractured food, which is missing an essential component - fiber. When we consume enough fiber, we take a load off of our organism by improving our elimination. Toxins often build up in the colon and

---

5 Kristine, "To Juice or Blend?" The Green Smoothie Community.
6 Wigmore, *Rebuild Your Health*.

fiber cleans them out. When most toxins have been removed by fiber, then the body has a greater ability to absorb nutrients, thus improving digestion. Humans could not live on juices alone, whereas green smoothies are a complete food."[7]

Victoria also did some excellent research that you may find worth reading in the "Blending vs. Juicing" which is excerpted on the Green Smoothie Revolution website. So, hopefully you now have a clearer understanding of what a green juice and a green smoothie are, how they differ and who should extract juices versus who should blend smoothies.

---

[7] Victoria Boutenko, "Blending vs. Juicing," Green Smoothie Revolution, December 1, 2009. http://greensmoothiesblog.com/blending-vs-juicing/.

2.

Green Smoothie Basics

Components: What's In A Green Smoothie?

Shortly after I gave birth to my daughter, I made an observation which led me to explore the world of Green Smoothies. Almost every week, I saw a friend posting on social media about some green juice or green smoothie that they had drank or wanted to try. At that time, I'd enjoyed a few myself and I could remember my introduction to the world of green beverages. It started with an extremely, refreshing bottle of Callaloo Juice that I had randomly picked up off a supermarket shelf some years before. That dark green blend of nourishment had only 5 ingredients: Water, Callaloo, Lime Juice, Ginger and Sugarcane Juice. In many ways, the original green smoothie has the same components as that bottle of the Callaloo beverage I enjoyed: liquid, green leaves, fruit and some extras (a medicinal herb, a flavourful spice and a natural sweetener). As explained earlier, a green smoothie is not a green juice nor a vegetable juice, but they may, as in this case, contain the same ingredients. In its purest form, a green smoothie is a creamy blend of green leaves, fruit and water – no strainers, no sweeteners.

Leaves

Dark, green leafy vegetables, greens, leafy greens, leafy veggies or green leaves are the essential component of every green smoothie. It is important to distinguish the leaves from other kinds of vegetables when talking about green smoothies. We may use any green leaves that we have in our kitchen, e.g. Callaloo (Green Amaranth), Lettuce, Cabbage or Pakchoy. So, there is no need to buy any imported, exotic 'super food'. Other leaves that can be blended into our green smoothies are: Broccoli, Cauliflower, Celery, Chinese Cabbage, Moringa, Kale and Spinach.

Fruits

Even the chimpanzees know that the best way to consume green leaves is to overpower the flavour with the natural sweetness of ripe fruits like Banana, Mango, Pineapple and Watermelon. Every kind of fruit is acceptable - even those that are not sweet (once we can tolerate it). The fruit can either be fresh or frozen , just ensure that they are fully ripened (because their primary purpose is to 'sweeten' the greens). The juicier the fruits, the better. Some easy to find and popular choices are Pawpaw, Orange, Otaheite Apple, Cherry, Lime and June Plum.

Liquids

In most cases, the water content of the fruits in a smoothie will not be sufficient for moving the ingredients around in the blender jar. As such, we should use carefully selected and 100% natural liquids to assist the blender blades in pulverising the leaves and chunks of fruit. The best choice is pure water, but if we want to add some variety and flavour, we may choose to use coconut water, 100% fruit juice, some herbal tea or a plant milk (like coconut milk or almond milk). But, don't use any pasteurised, sugar-added, artificially-flavoured, or carbonated liquids. Just keep it as simple and pure as possible.

Extras

Even the most basic of green smoothie recipes can be redesigned and re-purposed with the addition of one extra ingredient. Whether it is a herb that aids with detoxification, spices that enhance the flavours,   fillers that make the smoothie thick enough to serve as a meal replacement or sweeteners to give the extra energy and help the emerald-hued 'medicine' go down. Some fantastic herbs that are easy to find and very beneficial to include in green smoothies are: Mint, Thyme, Parsley, Basil, Sorrel and Rosemary. The spices that can put a kick in your glass include: Ginger, Cinnamon, Nutmeg, Vanilla and even Scotch Bonnet Pepper. Cashew Nuts, Peanut Butter, Oats and Flaxseeds serve as excellent fillers when you need that extra bulk; and the sweeteners we use should be as close to nature as possible, like Raisins, Sugarcane Juice, Molasses or Honey.

The 60/40 Rule: The Formula For Yumminess

The first false assumption that green smoothie newbies make, is that the blend needs to taste like liquefied bush, lawnmower pulp or some other bitter and unpleasant concoction. But, once they use a well developed recipe, they're bound to discover that green smoothies are delicious and very satisfying. Just like the chimpanzees that Victoria Boutenko had observed, we add fruit to our leaves to make eating them enjoyable. Just because dark, green leafy vegetables are good for you doesn't mean they need to taste yucky. This is why, for every blend of leafy greens and fruits we make, we follow the 60/40 rule. The 60:40 rule or 60/40 formula translates into recipes that call for blending a proportion of 60% fruits to 40% greens leaves each and every time. In this way, we ensure that when we drink a green smoothie, we taste the fruity flavours and not the greens.   In simple terms, this formula is telling us that we need to combine more fruits than greens when making a smoothie. Therefore, the ratio would work out to something like, 3 cups fruit to 2 cups leaves, and it is the perfect place to start for most persons.

It has been observed, that as we develop the habit of drinking a cup of green smoothie a day, our palate changes and we actually begin to enjoy the taste of leafy greens. As this happens, we'll start to feel as if the same recipes we've been blending for weeks, suddenly tastes a bit too sweet! When this happens, all we need to do is to increase the amount of leaves and decrease the amount of fruits we add to our smoothies. This will work out to something like a 70:30 ratio of leaves to fruits. Yet still, we do have a few persons who, because of their severe sweet tooth and heavy consumption of sugars, will find even the 60:40 ratio of fruit to leaves still to 'green' for their liking. If this is your experience, all you'll need to do is to adjust the recipe so that it looks more like

70% fruits to 30% leaves or just add some natural sweeteners until you acquire an appreciation for drinking up your leafy greens.

Creamy Fruits: The Key To The Perfect Emulsion

To be truly delightful in the mouth, a green smoothie needs to be thick and smooth. However, if you take just any, old random combination of leafy greens and fruit to make your green smoothie - while it may be tasty - may not result in the dreamy goodness that you want to enjoy. You just might end up with a green 'slushie' or 'sludgie' instead of a 'smoothie'. Different persons will give you different explanations as to why some smoothies come out creamier than others. However, my solution to the problem is to <u>always include at least 1 creamy fruit</u>. But, what are *creamy fruits* and what makes them worthy of being classified as such? The main method I use for identifying a creamy fruit from a watery or 'flavour' fruit, is by checking how much clear juice is produced when I squeeze the flesh of the fruit between my fingers. The most commonly used creamy fruit would be the Ripe Banana, and you will find that even the first green smoothie blended up by Victoria Boutenko, used Bananas. But, don't worry if you don't like or can't eat Bananas - you can leave them out. Just use a different creamy fruit in its place, since we still want that smooth creamy texture. Some other creamy fruits, which are great alternatives to Ripe Bananas, are Mangoes, (Avocado) Pears and Pawpaws.

The Four Types of Green Smoothies

We know that Victoria Boutenko's first green smoothie was a blend of Kale, Banana and Water - an authentic and very basic green smoothie. But, many fans of the green beverage have made their own variations and additions, to produce hundreds, if not thousands, of different green smoothie recipes, since then. Green smoothie blenders will notice the different purposes and recipe formulas used to make various of these blends, and I have classified four types of green smoothies based on their components and benefits:

1. Daily

This is the basic green smoothie that will become your daily habit, because the combinations are just pure and simple. It only contains leaves, fruit and water - just like Victoria's first green smoothie. The recipes may call for more than one type of leaves and more than one fruit, but only pure water, coconut water or natural fruit juices are used in them. These Daily Green Smoothies are the easiest and best to start with if your new to drinking green beverages.

2. Dessert

Even the most rigid of health enthusiasts gets the desire for something a little delectable every once in a while. These indulgent green smoothies combine leaves, fruit, plant milks, nuts or nut butters and natural sweeteners for a dessert-like treat. Dessert Green Smoothies are all-natural, healthful and guilt-free pleasures that you will enjoy for a weekend treat. They are great for children, serving up at dinner parties, or satisfying the momentary sweet-tooth.

3. Detox

These cleansing green smoothies are powered by the emulsion of leaves, fruit and unsweetened tea, supercharged with a blend of local herbs, fragrant spices and lots of citrus. The medicinal properties of the ingredients in these green beverages are designed to help the body eliminate toxins and to facilitate the body's natural healing processes in a gentler way. The herbal (bush) teas that are recommended include: Fever Grass, Sorrel, Cerasee and Peppermint for the beginners, and Moringa, Neem, Guinea Hen Weed and Bissy for those who have a more intimate knowledge of Jamaica's medicinal plants. All of these herbal teas may be purchased in commercially-packaged teabags, from local tea producers, which come with simple instructions for the novice. Citrus fruits (blended whole or juiced) are key components in a Detox Green Smoothie, just as much as healing spices like Ginger, Turmeric, Pimento and Cinnamon, when you're looking for a gentle, safe way to give your body a reboot.

4. Diet

Diet Green Smoothies are great as meal replacements and help to curb cravings for the weight-conscious. The high fibre content of these filling smoothies are reinforced by the inclusion of grains (whether raw, cooked or soaked), nuts, seeds and sweeteners that are added to the basic blend of leaves, fruit and water. Also known as Green Thickies, these blends that include all natural fillers like Oats, Peanut Butter, Pumpkin Seeds or Cashew Nuts will provide the right amount of bulk you need to keep your stomach full for longer. Often, twice the size of other green smoothies, Diet Green Smoothies allow you to fill up with nutrient dense calories and fat-fighting fibre to help you meet your weight loss goals.

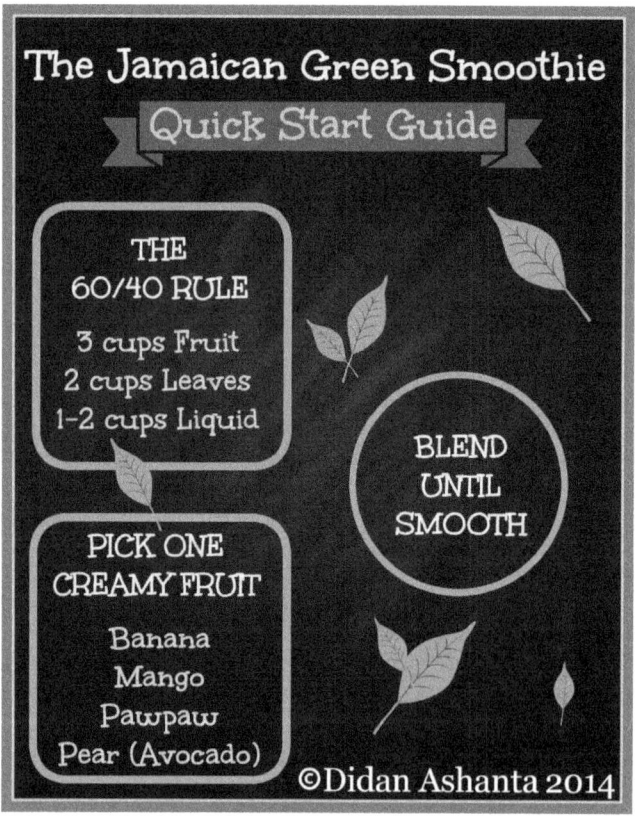

The Jamaican Green Smoothie
Quick Start Guide

THE
60/40 RULE

3 cups Fruit
2 cups Leaves
1-2 cups Liquid

BLEND
UNTIL
SMOOTH

PICK ONE
CREAMY FRUIT

Banana
Mango
Pawpaw
Pear (Avocado)

©Didan Ashanta 2014

3.

Green Smoothie Benefits

What Are the Benefits of Green Smoothies?

It is one thing to know what a green smoothie is and another thing to know how to make it, but why should anyone be gulping down the creamy, green stuff? Well, there are many benefits to gain from picking up a green smoothie habit. A quick spin around the internet will uncover story after story about how the addition of a daily green smoothie resulted in a life-transforming difference in the lives of countless persons. But, beyond the online hype and the testimonials from perfect strangers, there must be some science behind the liquefied nutritional package we're pouring out of our blenders. So, instead of posting more testimonials or a list of diseases and discomforts that have been alleviated or eliminated by the consistent consumption of green smoothies, let's take a look at the nutrition that's locked away inside our dark, green leafy vegetables.

Dietary Balance

We have all heard or read the phrase 'a balanced diet', but most people don't really know what that translates into as they eat their daily meals. The dietary guidelines that we use in the Caribbean, come in the form of the "Six Food Groups", and we are expected to eat a variety of foods, from each of the food groups, at each meal to have a balanced diet. When Jamaican students are being taught about food, nutrition and dietary requirements, these food groups are displayed on a piechart, which show the portions we should be eating from each food group. In the order from largest to smallest, the food groups are Staples, Legumes, Vegetables, Fruits, Food from Animals, and Fats & Oils. Yet, most of us never eat enough vegetables or fruits, and in some embarrassing cases, some of us eat no vegetable nor fruit at any of our mealtimes. Yet, it goes without saying that if we are to gain optimal nutrition for health and wellness, we must eat a balanced diet. It is from these foods, that we get the nutrients we need to maintain and improve our bodies and minds.

Increased Consumption of Fruit & Vegetables

The wonderful thing that a green smoothie allows us to do, is to easily and pleasantly increase the amount of fruits and vegetables we consume on a daily basis - without making any significant changes to the foods we already eat. A cup of green smoothie can become that plug that fits perfectly into the hole in our nutritional wall, because the amount of leafy greens and fruits we can get into a 16oz cup of green smoothie would equal 2 large salads. The difference is that it is so much easier to *drink* a vegetable salad and a fruit salad instead of trying to chew them both, in one go.

Just One Cup a Day

Nutritionists currently recommend that we include about 5 servings of fruit and vegetables in our meals every day. To be clear, one serving of leafy green veggies is about a cup and one serving of sliced up fruits would also equal a cup. For most persons, that would mean eating at least one fruit and one vegetable in every meal, and although that isn't an impossible feat, very few people are doing it. *Are you?* Well, not to worry if you aren't, because we can easily meet our daily requirements for fruits and vegetables by drinking *just one cup* of green smoothie a day! That's because green smoothies allow us to stuff a fruit salad and a veggie salad into our blenders and drink up loads of nutrient-dense, delicious creaminess with no hassle.

Daily Habit

All we need to do is to make a habit of drinking a green smoothie everyday. Once you start your day with a green smoothie, you can rest assured that you have had your daily requirement of fruits and vegetables and not need to worry about what you eat for the rest of the day. By drinking a green smoothie a day, you would be free of guilt and worry and you would be feeling good about eating or *drinking* right. With the average omnivorous diet, one usually gets enough Carbohydrates, Proteins and Fats to meet and even exceed the recommended daily intake. But, only a high consumption of plant-foods like fruits and leafy green vegetables can completely account for the recommended daily intake of Vitamins, Minerals, Water and Dietary Fibre. So, if you can't think of any other reason to make a cup of green smoothie a daily habit, then do it for the sake of a feeding your body a balanced diet.

Dietary Fibre, Health & Wellness

By consuming green smoothies, your body will be forced to process a larger amount of dietary fibre (also known as 'roughage') than it has been accustomed to. This increase in your fibre intake will result in an initial few days of bloating, gassiness, more frequent bowel movements and even softer stool. But these are all natural reactions of the digestive system to dietary fibre. The reason this will happen is because your body has been deprived of an adequate supply of this very important nutrient, and by drinking green smoothies, you are creating a sudden flood of 'fibrosity' that will be a surprise to both you and your digestive system. The key to handling this digestive 'culture shock' is by sustaining - *not stopping* - your intake of high quantities of plant foods (e.g. green smoothies), and more importantly, by increasing the amount of water you drink everyday.

Water & Dietary Fibre

Why more water? Well, imagine that you have a drain that has been plugged up with gunk and sludge and you're having trouble with the blockage and yucky stuff is backing up in your sink. You would have to use a scouring pad or steel-wire brush to dislodge the gunk and sludge from the sides of the drain, and then you would probably pour some grease-cutting chemicals in there, as well. Well, dietary fibre exists in two forms, as soluble fibre and insoluble fibre. The insoluble fibre is like the scouring pad, which bulks up and pushes waste matter and bacteria quickly through our digestive system. While the soluble fibre dissolves in water and is gelatinous, so it acts like the grease-cutting chemicals by moving through our intestines slowly. The soluble fibre also ferments and creates gases that move the waste and toxic substances out of our bodies. Yet, both soluble and insoluble fibre need water to complete their work in the digestive process.

The soluble fibre needs to be dissolved in water and the insoluble fibre needs to absorb the water. So, in the case of the blocked up drain, if you don't flood the drain with lots of water, the gunk, sludge and chemicals will simply pile up inside the passage and even worsen the blockage. In our digestive system, we call that 'constipation'. This is why drinking large quantities of water is important. It will help to flush out waste matter, increase the elimination of bacteria and toxic substances, soften our stool and make our bowel movements more frequent. Therefore, when you start your green smoothie habit, as soon as you begin to sense the changes in your body, (whether they are feelings of gassiness or more frequent bowel movements) please try to double whatever quantities of water you usually drink on a daily basis - until you average about 2-3 litres for the day. By increasing your fluid intake, you are helping the body to flush out the longstanding build up of waste matter, bacteria and toxins that has been sitting in your intestines and colon for ages. In fact, your body's ability to eliminate waste material, bacteria and toxic substances, is key to your overall health and well-being. So, green smoothies or not, we need to keep hydrated.

Detoxification & Disease Prevention

Medical professionals will explain that the body detoxifies (eliminates toxic substances) naturally when we exhale, perspire, urinate and defecate. Yet, most of us are not living lifestyles that allow our lungs, skins, kidneys, livers and colons to do their jobs effectively and efficiently. We spend our in days in air-conditioned buildings and vehicles, and our streets are filled will exhaust and noxious fumes. Then when it comes to what we put into our bodies, pure water, fresh fruits and vegetables do not account for half of the things we consume daily. But, how can we perspire, urinate and defecate sufficiently if we don't put right foods and beverages in our bodies for optimal elimination? We already know that a toxic colon is, unfortunately, the cause of a lot of chronic disease. After all, our parents and grandparents have been staunch advocates and enforcers of the "washout"! Whether it was a dose of Brooklax, Epsom salts, Sulphur bitters, Aloe juice, Castor oil or some bush (herbal) tea, according to the old folks: almost all ailments could be resolved by a good 'washout'.

In addition to cleaning out our guts, a diet that is high in fibre is proven to extend our lives by lowering our risks for chronic, lifestyle-related illnesses like heart disease, diabetes, obesity, high cholesterol and hypertension, among others. The connection between fibre, digestion, detoxification and wellness is based on how the body handles waste. If any of the waste elimination organs or systems fail to function or becomes overloaded, the work of eliminating the excess waste is passed on to the other organs or systems. If these systems become overloaded, as well, then the body begins to absorb the waste and bacteria resulting in toxicity, which manifests itself as disease. This process only highlights the importance of an efficiently functioning digestive system; and since we can't get any fibre from eating animal products (chicken, fish, beef, pork, mutton, milk, cheese, yogurt, eggs), we have to ensure that we get a hearty serving of fruits and vegetables everyday.

Chlorophyll: Liquid Sunshine

But, you may ask, "Why leafy greens and not just any vegetable?" Well, that's because leafy greens contain the 'green blood of plants' also known as *chlorophyll*, which is a green pigment found within the *leaves* of plants. Now, we know that people and animals eat food to get energy, and that most of the food that people and animals eat comes from plants, for example, corn, oranges, peanuts, and, yams. But, plants create their own food through photosynthesis. During this process, plants absorb light energy from the sun (the earth's ultimate life/energy source) through their leaves and the chlorophyll in the leaves traps the energy which the plant converts into a carbohydrate (sugar). It is this photosynthesised food that the plant uses for nourishment, respiration (producing oxygen) and growth. As such, when we blend leafy greens in our smoothies, we break into the cells of the leaves and gain access to this *liquid sunshine*: chlorophyll.

Nutrient Rich & Nutrient Quick

If you were to check the nutritional supplement stock at your local pharmacy or health food store, you may be surprised to find *liquid chlorophyll* being sold for a wide range of health benefits, particularly as it relates to our blood. That's because the molecular structure of chlorophyll is almost identical to the molecular structure of haemoglobin - with the only difference being that chlorophyll has magnesium at its core, while haemoglobin has iron at its core. But, instead of purchasing a shelf-stable nutritional supplement, we can get fresh and un-manipulated chlorophyll by blending up a daily cup of green smoothies. The presence of dark, green leaves in our smoothies allows us to flood our bodies with various key nutrients because greens are rich in vitamins A, C, E and K, many B vitamins, and antioxidants. Dark, green leafy vegetables are also great sources of iron, magnesium, potassium and calcium. So, by consuming hearty servings of leafy greens every day, we enable our bodies to protect our cells and prevent cancer development in the colon, lung, breast and cervix. By drinking green smoothies, we can promote heart health, build and maintain strong bones and muscles, stabilise our blood pressure and help with the proper clotting of blood.

Quick Absorption

Yet, with all these benefits sitting in a bunch of leafy greens, salads still fail to make frequent appearances during most mealtimes and even simple stir-fries are not the traditional main dish. Aside from the boring way in which most leafy greens are prepared for eating, most of us are not keen on spending the time nor making the effort required to thoroughly chew our food. But, a reputable medical professional or nutritional expert would inform you that we need to chew our food until it is completely liquefied in our mouths for our bodies to access the optimum nutritional benefits. This is why blending dark, green leafy vegetables into green smoothies is the easiest and most efficient way to flush our organ systems with all these vitamins, minerals and antioxidants; and also the reason we will benefit from drinking green smoothies in many ways, including:

- Improved Digestion

- Waste Elimination Regularity

- Weight Loss

- Decreased Cravings

- Improved Blood Circulation

- Glowing Skin

- Immunity Boost

- Increased Energy

- Mental Clarity

- Better Sleep

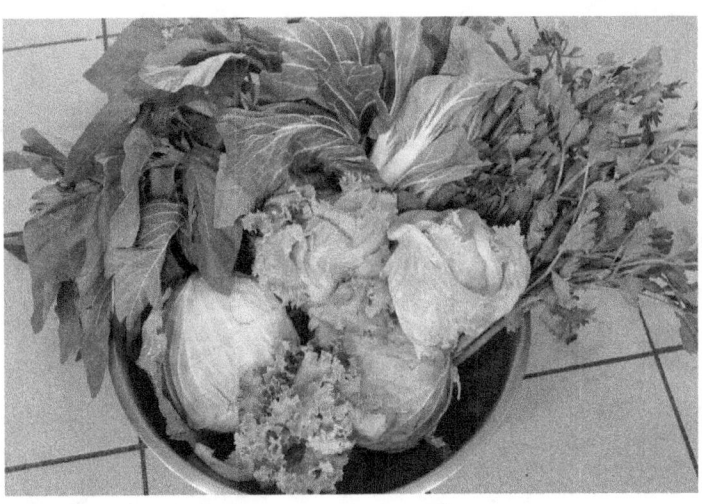

4.

Leafy Green Hazards

Anti-nutrients & Toxicity

Now, that you have caught a snapshot of some of the benefits of developing a green smoothie habit, you may still have a hard time shaking the nagging question about the hazards of drinking liquefied leafy greens. "Won't drinking green smoothies be harmful to my health?", you ask. You will probably even show me an article or two that you've come across, that warns about 'oxalates' and 'alkaloids'. Well, I'm glad you've brought up the topic, because in every area of life it is always important that we maintain a balance; as ultimately, we don't want to be guilty of consuming 'too much of a good thing', right? So, I'll go right ahead and answer your question: No, drinking green smoothies is <u>not</u> harmful to your health. But, poor eating and farming habits are! By 'poor eating habits', I'm referring to the practice of binging on a limited amount of foods. For optimal nutrition, we must always try to eat a wide variety of foods. So, by diversifying our diet, our bodies can benefit from a broader spectrum of nutrients; and we can avoid anti-nutrient toxicity. A diversified diet is essential because all foods, even within the same group (for example, berries or leaves), contain different types and quantities of vitamins, minerals and phytochemicals; and by eating various foods, we allow our bodies to benefit from a more comprehensive supply of nutrients. Anti-nutrient toxicity is a possibility since the types and quantities of anti-nutrients (compounds found in foods and beverages that interfere with the absorption of vitamins, minerals or phytochemicals) will vary from plant to plant. As such, a heavily-restricted and overly limited diet is dangerous to our health and well-being.

So, why have some persons issued warnings about leafy greens? Well, we know that some animals are herbivores (e.g. rabbits, cattle, horses, elephants, and goats) and they get their food from plants only without facing any problems with anti-nutrient toxicity. This is because herbivores are grazers or foragers, meaning they eat whatever they find in one location and then move on to another location to eat whatever they find there. This means that the plants from which they have eaten will get a chance for their leaves and fruits to grow back; and if the animal eats fruits from those plants, the seeds from those fruits will be spread to other locations through the animal's droppings. Human beings, on the other hand, have decided that it is better to stay in one location, forever, eating the plants (and animals) that they have nearby. But, if we were to select only one leafy green vegetable, and decide that it is the ultimate source of all nutrition and eat it everyday, eventually all of those plants would be wiped out! Or, even become the source of multinational wars. So, Nature's wisdom included alkaloids in leafy greens to serve as the plants' defence against extinction, and to encourage us to eat a variety of foods, from all the food groups everyday. However, please make a note that dark, green leafy vegetables are not the only source of anti-nutrients in our diet - herbivore or not. The following naturally-occurring chemical compounds are some of the most frequently referenced when talking about alkaloids in dark green, leafy vegetables:

• Goitrogen - also found in Peanuts, Strawberries and Sweet Potatoes.

• Oxalic Acid - also found in Cassava, Garlic and String Beans.

• Oxalate - also found in Nuts, Chocolate and Black Pepper.

Moderation & Rotation

So, what should we do to ensure that our green smoothie habit doesn't become hazardous and toxic? We should practise moderation and rotation. By consuming all our greens in moderation we are able to minimise the amount of anti-nutrients that can build up in our organ systems. Therefore, just because we have learnt about the benefits of consuming dark green, leafy vegetables and since we have recognised that green smoothies are the easiest and most efficient way of consuming enough greens, we should not run out and adopt a diet that is exclusively comprised of greens! We have to take all good things in moderation; plus, we must not forget about *nutrient variation*. So, while we may decide to add a cup of green smoothie to our regular daily meals, we will only get optimal benefits from using different types of greens, from the different plant families. Yes, I said, 'plant families'. Not all leafy green veggies are created equal (*smile*); and although it is not necessary to become expertly familiar with the various plant families in order to rotate your greens, it may help to become acquainted with how they are grouped as you try to rotate and vary your greens. These are the most common plant families for the dark, green leafy vegetables that we use to make green smoothies:

- Brassicaceae e.g. Pakchoy, Cabbage, Kale.

- Amaranthaceae e.g. Callaloo, Spinach.

- Asteraceae e.g. Lettuce, Dandelion.

- Apiaceae e.g. Parsley, Celery.

By looking at this listing, we can get an idea of which greens are in the same family, and as such, would supply similar nutritional packages and therefore try to avoid blending our green smoothies from only one family of plants. Yet, while a little knowledge is empowering, I would not recommend becoming obsessed with the technicalities and 'science' behind rotating your greens, because our bodies are quite capable of absorbing what is needed and eliminating the excess. Plus, if we eat according to the seasons and according to which produce is in abundance, then Nature will effortlessly cause us to rotate and moderate. Just think about how so many of us grew up eating Callaloo for breakfast almost everyday when the garden was full of plump bundles ready for harvest. Or, how almost every lunch shop serves shredded Cabbage as the side salad in their boxed lunches, when the market was flooded with cheap, leafy heads. None of that 'excessive' daily consumption of these leafy green vegetables have been shown to cause harm to any of us. So, don't get too carried away or legalistic about the matter of rotation among plant families.

Wild & Uncommon Edibles

But, if you really grow concerned about the variety of leafy greens that you have available to you, or you get bored with the variety that is in abundance, there is an endless supply of wild and uncommon edible leaves that may be used for your daily green smoothie. The leaves of many of the fruits and vegetables that we eat on a daily basis are also edible and would serve us well if blended in a green smoothie, instead of being trashed. Some examples are the leaves from Cassava and Coco tubers, Otaheite Apple and Pawpaw trees, or even the tops of Turnips, Beetroots and Carrots. Other dark, green leafy vegetables that are edible and may be used to make our green smoothies are the leaves from the Dasheen, Yam, Sweet Potato, and Pumpkin plants. Yet, even though all these leaves are edible, they are rarely used for food in Jamaica, because most people place no nutritional nor economical value on them. This means that you may be able to acquire these wild and uncommon edibles quite cheaply, if not freely from your neighbours, local farmers or even your favourite market vendor. The leaves of the Moringa tree are currently a popular wild edible that you may want to try, as well as the leaves of the Purslane plant, that grows wild in many Jamaican yards and is often discarded as a weed. Some persons blend the Moringa leaves fresh from their backyard, while others put them to dry and grind them to a powder, which they toss into green smoothies as an 'extra'.

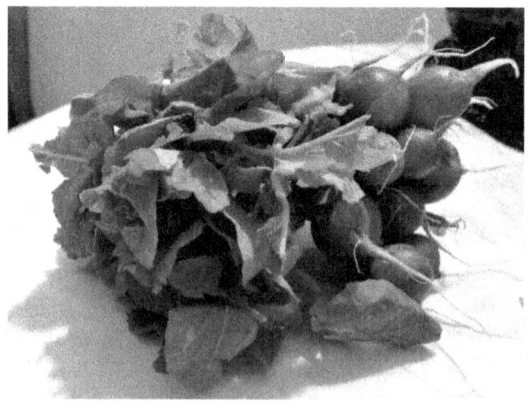

Pesticides

A poor farming habit that may seriously affect your health, while drinking green smoothies, is the use of synthetic pesticides. If you have ever grown a bundle of Callaloo in your backyard garden, then you know that we don't need to use synthetic pesticides to harvest quality produce. But, many commercially grown leafy greens have been treated with these chemicals and may have pesticide residue on them, even after being reaped and packaged for sale. So, by eating foods (even fruits and other vegetables) that have been treated by these harmful chemicals, you are exposing your body to high levels of toxicity.

Pesticides in food can build up in the body, disable the body's immune system and retard the body's waste elimination organ systems and detoxification mechanisms. The habit of blending leafy greens and fruits into green smoothies definitely helps us to consume larger quantities of produce and allows our bodies to absorb more nutrients than just casual chewing. However, this high nutrient potency from a consuming liquefied foods also comes with potential dangers: if the produce (both fruits and leafy greens) are have pesticide residue on.

Just in the same way that liquefying the food floods our bodies with nutrients, if the produce is still coated with harmful chemicals, we are effectively consuming and absorbing larger quantities of the chemicals than we would if they were not liquefied. So, it is very important that as we select produce for our daily green smoothies, we take the necessary precautions to ensure they are free from chemical pesticides.

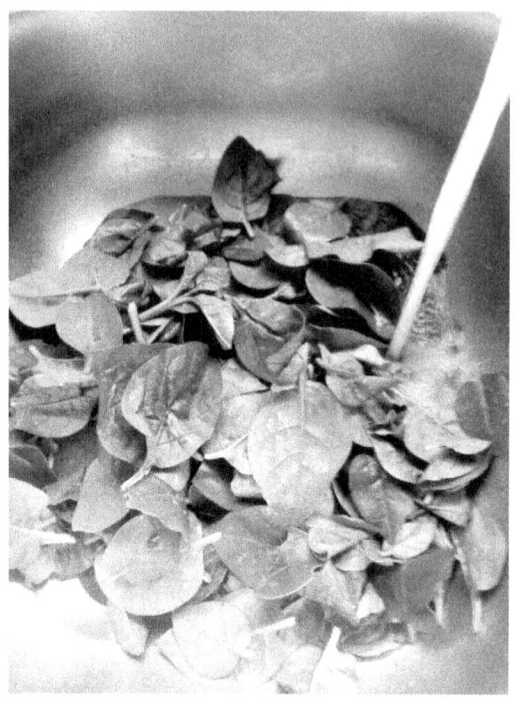

If you can't avoid conventionally-grown produce, please be careful to thoroughly wash and lightly scrub your fruits. Soak your leafy greens in a vinegar solution (1 part vinegar to 2 parts water); or fill a basin/kitchen sink with water and about 1/4 cup of hydrogen peroxide, soak the leafy greens in the solution for about 20 minutes, then rinse in running water and pat dry. But, the best preventative step, for avoiding pesticide build up, is to grow your produce; and if you can't grow it, choose organic produce.

5.

Jamaican Green Smoothie Recipes

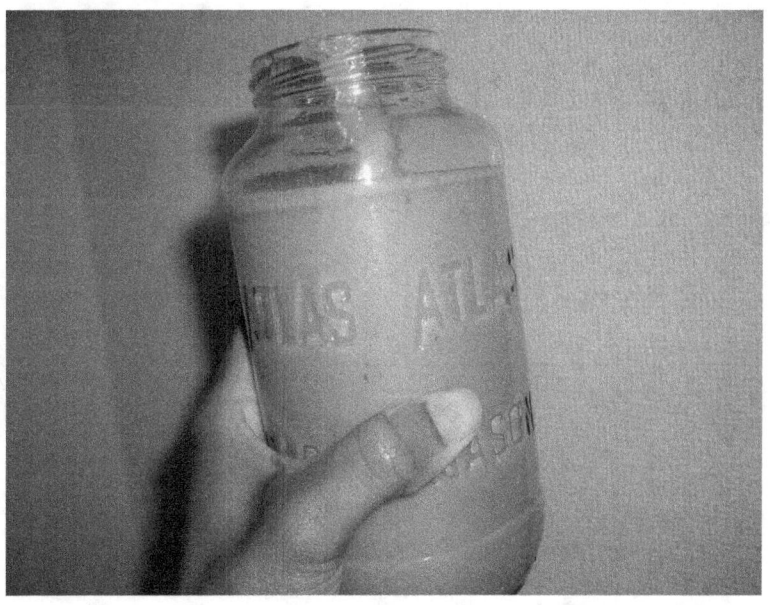

**Please Note: You may use ANY dark, green leafy
vegetable to make these green smoothies!**

The leafy greens listed in the following recipes are just an
indication of the wide variety of locally-grown produce available in
Jamaica. So, please feel free to use whichever greens you have in
your backyard as you enjoy these blends.

Daily: Basic Blends For Your Everyday Habit

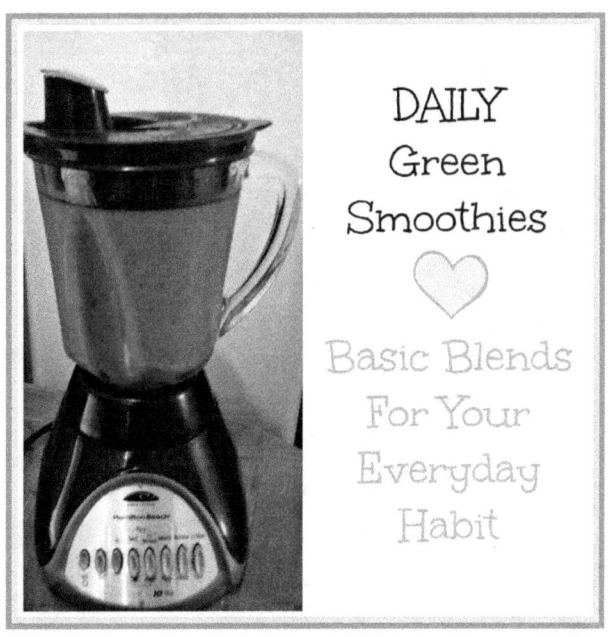

Mango Walk

<u>Ingredients</u>

2 Cups Spinach, chopped

1-2 Cups Water

3 Cups Mango, chopped

1 Lime, juiced

<u>Method</u>

Blend the Spinach and Water until all the leaves are finely shredded.

Add the Mango chunks and Lime Juice, and blend until smooth.

Purple Passion

<u>Ingredients</u>

2 Cups Pakchoy, chopped

1-2 Cups Coconut Water

1 Cup Ripe Banana, sliced

2 Cups Otaheite Apple, chopped

<u>Method</u>

Blend the Callaloo and Coconut Water until all the leaves are finely shredded.

Add the Banana and Apple, then blend until smooth.

Jamaica Sweet

Ingredients

2 Cups Radish Leaves

1-2 Cups Water

1 Cup Ripe Banana, chopped

2 Cup Sweetsop, de-seeded

1 Lime, juiced

Method

Blend the Radish Leaves in the Water until no bits are visible.

Add the Banana, Sweetsop and Lime Juice, then blend until smooth.

Sweet Sapphire

Ingredients

2 Cups Kale

1-2 Cups Coconut Water

1 Cup Pawpaw

2 Cups Jackfruit pegs

1 Tsp Ginger, minced

Method

Liquefy the Kale in the Coconut Water.

Add the Pawpaw, Jackfruit and minced Ginger, then blend until smooth.

Emerald Sunrise

<u>Ingredients</u>

2 Cups Baby Bokchoy

1 Cup Orange Juice, freshly squeezed

2 Cups Ripe Banana

2 Cups Pineapple, chopped

<u>Method</u>

Blend the Baby Bokchoy in the Orange Juice until liquefied.

Add the Banana and Pine, then blend until smooth.

Berry Cooler

Ingredients

2 Cups Watercress

1 Cup Water

1 Cup Ripe Banana

1 Cup Cucumber

1 Cup Strawberries

1 Tsp Ginger, minced

Method

Blend the Watercress in the Water until all the leaves are finely shredded.

Add the fruits and minced Ginger, then blend until smooth.

Da 9-inch Wine

Ingredients

2 Cups Romaine Lettuce

1-2 Cups Water

2 Cup Ripe Banana

1 Cups Naseberries, de-seeded

1 Lime, juiced

Method

Blend the Lettuce and Water until no bits are visible.

All the Naseberry, Banana and Lime Juice, then blend until smooth.

Guava-Pine Tumble

<u>Ingredients</u>

2 Cups Arugula (Rocket)

1-2 Cups Water

1 Cup Ripe Banana

1 Cup Guava

1 Cup Pineapple

<u>Method</u>

Liquefy the Arugula in the Water.

Add the fruits and blend until smooth.

Passion Statement

<u>Ingredients</u>

2 Cups Moringa Leaves

1-2 Cups Water

2 Cups Ripe Banana

1 Cup Passionfruit (pulp)

1 Lime, juiced

<u>Method</u>

Liquefy the Moringa in the Water.

Add the Banana, Passionfruit and Lime Juice, then blend until smooth.

Easy Morning

Ingredients

2 Cups Spinach, chopped

1-2 Cups Water

2 Cups Ripe Banana, sliced

1 Cup Pineapple, chopped

1 Lime, juiced

Method

Blend the Spinach and Water until no bits are visible.

Add the fruits and Lime Juice and blend until smooth.

Dessert: Indulgent Blends For Your Weekend Treat

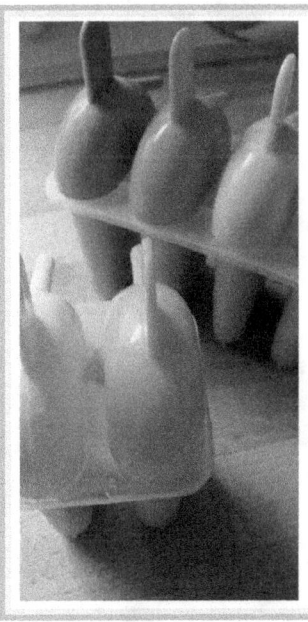

DESSERT
Green
Smoothies

Indulgent
Blends For
Your
Weekend
Treat

Nutty Mango MOUSSE

Ingredients

2 Cups Pakchoy

2/3-1 Cup Coconut Water

1 Cup Pear (Avocado)

2 Cups Mango, frozen

1/2 Cup Granola

Method

Liquefy the Pakchoy in the Coconut Water.

Add the Pear, Mango and Granola, and blend until smooth.

Serve in a bowl and eat with a spoon.

Substitution

You may use Grapenut Cereal instead of the Granola.

Merry Sunday MOUSSE

Ingredients

2 Cups Spinach

2/3-1 Cup Coconut Milk

1 Cup Soursop Pulp

2 Cups Pear (Avocado)

2 Tsp Sorrel Preserves

Method

Liquefy the Spinach in the Coconut Milk.

Add the Soursop, Pear and Sorrel Preserves, and blend until smooth.

Serve in a bowl and eat with a spoon.

Substitution

You may use Sorrel Jam or Jelly instead of the Sorrel Preserves.

Guava-Pinealloo ICE DREAM

Ingredients

2 Cups Callaloo Leaves

1 Cup Full-Fat Coconut Milk, chilled

1 Cup Ripe Banana, frozen

1 Cup Guava, frozen

1/2 Cup Pineapple, frozen

1 Tsp Raisins (optional)

1 Tsp Vanilla (optional)

Method

Blend the Callaloo and Coconut Milk until no bits are visible.

Add the frozen fruit, Raisins and Vanilla, then blend until smooth.

Enjoy as soft serve right away.

For Firmer Consistency

Place the ice cream in an airtight container in the freezer for 30 minutes.

Matrimony ICE DREAM

<u>Ingredients</u>

1 Cup Romaine Lettuce

1 Cup Full-Fat Coconut Milk, frozen into cubes

2 Cups Starapple, frozen

1 Cup Orange Segments

1/2 Tsp Nutmeg

1 Tsp Lime Juice

<u>Method</u>

Blend the Lettuce, Lime Juice and Orange Segments until liquefied.

Add the Starapple, Coconut Milk and Nutmeg, then blend until smooth.

Enjoy as soft serve right away.

<u>For Firmer Consistency</u>

Place the ice cream in an airtight container in the freezer for 30 minutes.

Skip-A-Round ICICLE

Ingredients

1 1/2 Cups Spinach

1/4 Cup Cherry Juice

2 Otaheite Apples

2 tbsp Honey (optional)

Method

Blend Spinach in Cherry Juice until no bits are visible.

Add Apples and Honey, then blend until smooth.

Pour the smoothie into icicle moulds and freeze.

Enjoy with the kids!

Minty Melon Slush ICICLE

Ingredients

2 Cups Callaloo Leaves

1-2 Cups Mint Tea

1 Cup Pear (Avocado)

2 Cups Watermelon, de-seeded

1 Lime, juiced

Method

Blend the Callaloo in the Mint Tea, until no bits are visible.

Add Pear, Watermelon and Lime Juice, and blend until smooth.

Pour the smoothie into icicle moulds, then freeze.

Enjoy with the kids!

Honeydew Colada COCKTAIL

Ingredients

2 Cups Spinach

1-2 Cups Coconut Milk

2 Cups Honeydew Melon

1 Cup Pineapple Chunks

1 Lime, juiced

Method

Blend the Spinach and Coconut Milk together until all the leaves are finely shredded.

Add the Honeydew, Pine and Lime Juice, then blend into an emulsion.

Sip slowly from your favourite cocktail glass.

Mean Salad COCKTAIL

Ingredients

2 Cups Pakchoy

1-2 Cups Coconut Water

1 Cup Mango Chunks

1 Cup Starapple, de-seeded

1/2 Cup Pineapple Chunks

1/2 Cup Orange Segments

Method

Blend the Pakchoy and Coconut Water together until liquefied.

Add the fruits, then blend into an emulsion.

Sip slowly from your favourite cocktail glass.

Detox: Cleansing Blends For Your One-Week Reboot

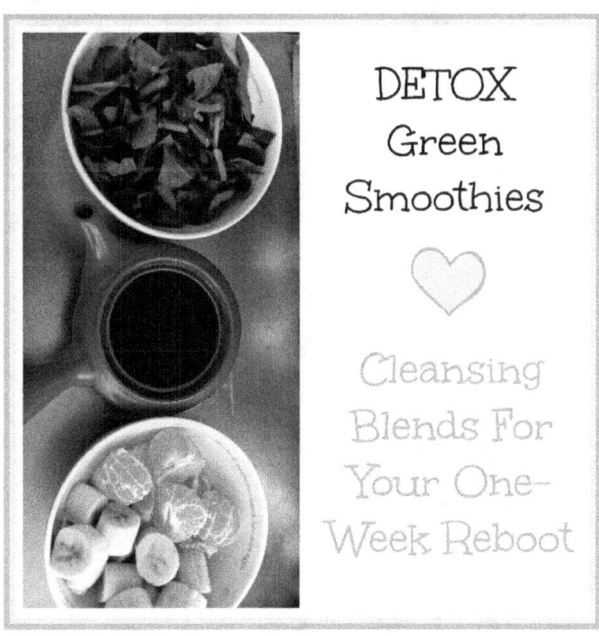

DETOX
Green
Smoothies

Cleansing
Blends For
Your One-
Week Reboot

Clean Scrub

Ingredients

2 Cups Purslane

2 Cups Coconut Water

2 Cup Pear (Avocado)

1 Cup Pawpaw

2 Tsp Ginger, minced

Method

Liquefy the Purslane in the Coconut Water.

Add the Pear, Pawpaw and Ginger, then blend until smooth.

Greenilious

<u>Ingredients</u>

2 Cups Pakchoy

2 Cups Grapefruit Juice

2 Cups Pear (Avocado)

1 Cup Ripe Banana

1 Lime, juiced

<u>Method</u>

Blend the Pakchoy and Grapefruit Juice until no bits are visible.

Add the Pear , Banana and Lime Juice, then blend until smooth.

Pull... Up!

<u>Ingredients</u>

1 Cup Mustard Greens

1 Cup Celery

1-2 Cups Ortanique Juice, freshly squeezed

2 Cups Pawpaw

1 Cup Mango

1 Tsp Ginger, minced

<u>Method</u>

Liquefy the leaves in the Ortanique Juice.

Add the fruits and minced Ginger, then emulsify.

Pure Heart

<u>Ingredients</u>

2 Cups Spinach

1-2 Cups Cerasee Tea

2 Cups Mango

1 Cup Pineapple

1 Lime, juiced

<u>Method</u>

Blend the Spinach and Cerasee together, until all the leaves are finely shredded.

Add the fruits and Lime Juice, and blend into a smooth emulsion.

Back-to-School

Ingredients

2 Cups Callaloo Leaves

1-2 Cups Aloe Juice

1 Cup Pawpaw

1 Ripe Banana

2 Tangerines

Method

Blend the Callaloo in the Aloe Juice until liquefied.

Add the Pawpaw, Banana and Tangerine, then blend until smooth.

Simmer Down

<u>Ingredients</u>

2 Cups Callaloo Leaves

1-2 Cups Fevergrass Tea

1 Cup Pear (Avocado)

2 Cups Pawpaw

1 Tsp Ginger, minced

1/2 Tsp Cinnamon Powder

<u>Method</u>

Blend the Callaloo in the Fevergrass Tea until liquefied.

Add the Pear, Pawpaw, Ginger and Cinnamon Powder, then blend until smooth.

Moringa Zinger

Ingredients

2 Cups Moringa Leaves

2 Cups Grapefruit Juice, freshly squeezed

3 Ripe Bananas

Method

Liquefy the Moringa Leaves in the Grapefruit Juice.

Add the Bananas and blend until smooth.

Diet: Filling Blends For Your Weight Loss Plan

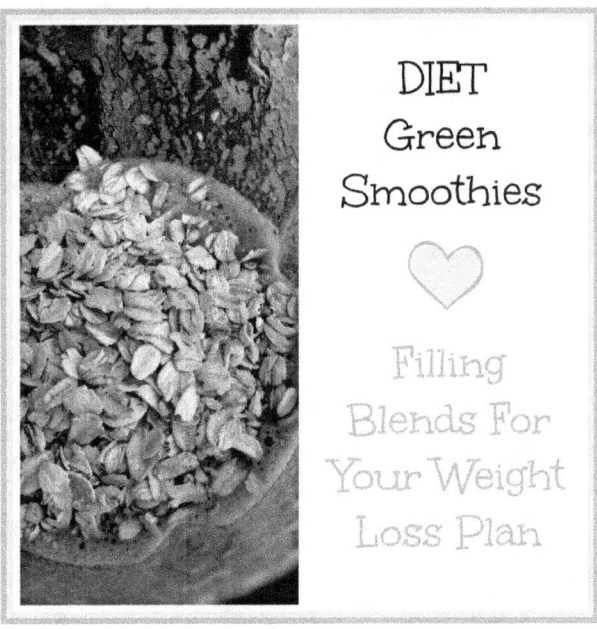

DIET
Green
Smoothies

Filling
Blends For
Your Weight
Loss Plan

Sunshine Thickie

Ingredients

1 Cup Romaine Lettuce

2 Cups Coconut Water

1 Cup Pawpaw

1 Cup Pineapple

1 Cup Oats (soaked, overnight)

Method

Liquefy the Lettuce in the Coconut Water.

Add the Pawpaw, Pine and Oats, then blend until smooth.

Golden Desire

<u>Ingredients</u>

2 Cups Baby Bok Choy

1 Sprig Mint Leaves

1-2 Cups Almond Milk

2 Cups Mango, chopped (frozen)

3 Passion Fruits (pulp)

<u>Method</u>

Blend the Callaloo, Mint and Coconut Milk until all the leaves are finely shredded.

Add the Mango and Passion, then blend until smooth.

Mango Melon Mash

Ingredients

3 Cups Watermelon, de-seeded

2 Cups Kale

1 Cup Oats (soaked overnight)

1 Cup Mango

1 Lime, juiced

Method

Blend the Watermelon and Kale until all the leaves are finely shredded.

Add the Oats, Mango and Lime Juice, then blend until smooth.

Tropical Tumble

<u>Ingredients</u>

2 Cups Pakchoy

2 Cups Water

1 Cup Pawpaw

1 Cup Guava

1 Cup Pineapple

<u>Method</u>

Blend the Pakchoy and Water together until no bits are visible.

Add the Pawpaw, Guava and Pine, then blend until smooth.

Passionate Punch

<u>Ingredients</u>

2 Cups Callaloo Leaves

2 Cups Coconut Milk

1 Cup Peanuts

2 Cups Mango

<u>Method</u>

Liquefy the Peanuts in the Coconut Milk.

Add the Callaloo and blend until no bits are visible.

Then, add the Mango and blend until smooth.

6.

Bonus Recipes - The Celebrity Gourmet Feature

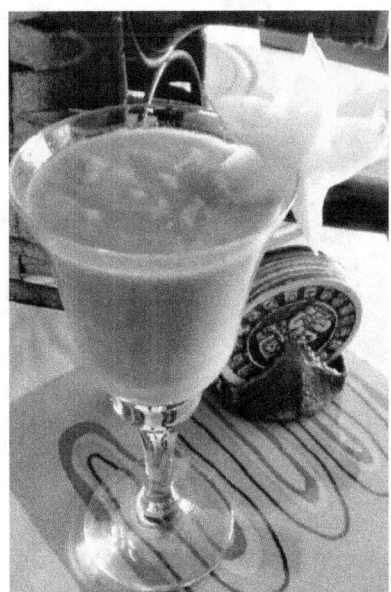

These wonderful recipes were graciously shared with me by some of Jamaica's favourite faces and household names. We hope that you'll enjoy these blends as much as they do.

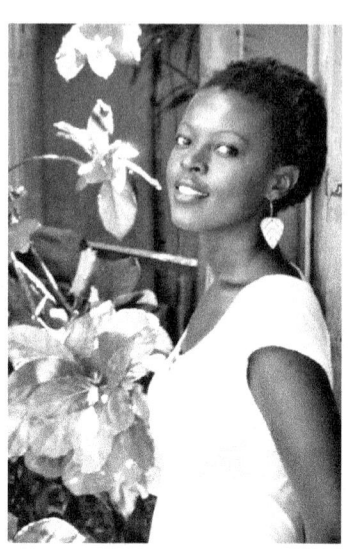

Bena Nakawuki

Live Food & Holistic Health Expert

Bena's Tropical Green Smoothie

Excellent for breakfast!

Ingredients

1 Handful of Spinach

1 Banana, frozen chunks

1/2 Cup Pineapple, chunks

1 Cup Almond Milk

1 Cup Cane Juice (Optional)

1/4 Tsp Cinnamon

1 Tsp Natural Vanilla Extract

1 Tbsp Coconut Oil (Cold-pressed)

Method

Put all ingredients into a blender. Start with 1 cup Almond Milk and add more, if necessary (to your desired consistency). Blend well, serve in a glass and enjoy.

Substitution

You may use Coconut Milk instead of Almond Milk.

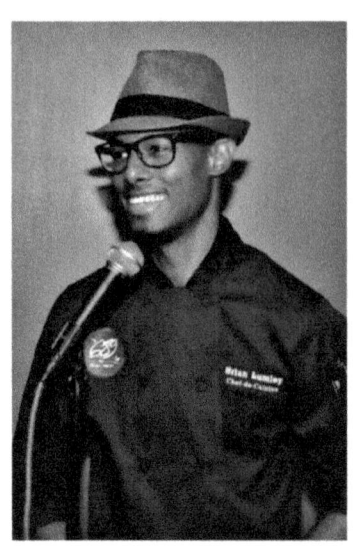

Brian Lumley

Chef & Owner of 689 by Brian Lumley

Chef Lumley's Starter Smoothie

Ingredients

2 Cups Fresh Spinach

2 Cups Water

1 Cup Pineapple

1 Cup Mango

2 Bananas

Method

Tightly pack your leafy greens into a measuring cup and toss into blender. Add water and blend together until all leafy chunks are gone. Next add in mango, pineapple and bananas (if used) and blend again.

Serves 2

Substitutions

You may use Callaloo instead of the Spinach. You may use an extra 1 cup of Mango instead of the Banana.

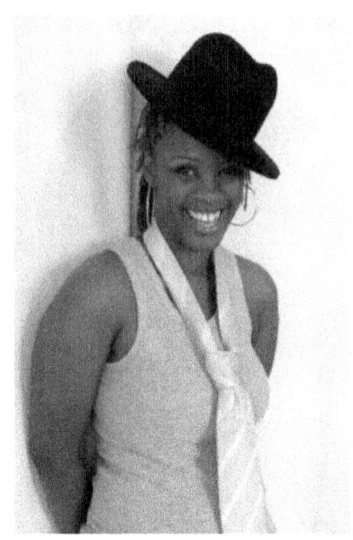

Simone
Camaley
Hamilton

Singer

Camaley's Sunrise Thickie

Ingredients

1 Cup Callaloo

1 Cup Pakchoy

1 Cup Banana

1 Cup Papaya

1 Cup Pineapple

1 Cup Coconut Water

1 Cup Almonds

Method

Soak the almonds overnight and chop the leaves and fruits for easy blending. Blend the Almonds in the Coconut water until liquefied then add the leaves and blend until no bits are visible. Add the fruits and blend until smooth.

Substitutions

You may use Water in the place of Coconut Water. Flaxseeds, Pumpkin Seeds (or other nuts or seeds of your choice) may be used instead of Almonds.

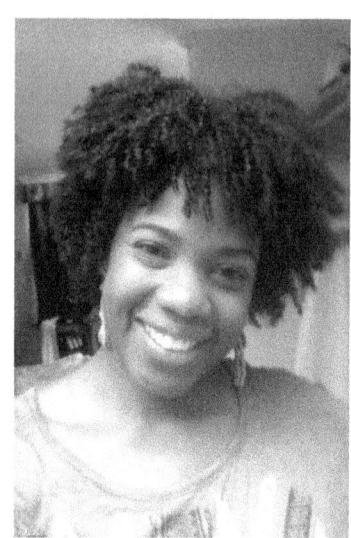

Cherie
Dowdie

Owner of
Live Juice
Bar

Cherie's Yummy Green Jackfruit Smoothie

Ingredients

2 Cups Jackfruit

1 1/2 Cups Pineapple Juice

2 Cups Leafy Greens of your choice

1/2 Tsp Pure Vanilla Extract

Method

Remove the seeds, membranes and strings from the Jackfruit.

Chop or rip the Leafy Greens. Add the Jackfruit and Leafy Greens to the blender and pour enough Pineapple Juice to cover.

Blend to desired smoothness. Add remaining Pineapple Juice and Vanilla Extract. Add ice if desired, or chill before serving.

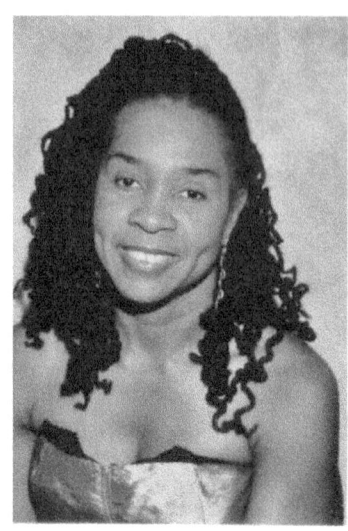

Cheryl
Holdsworth

Educator
& Owner of
Cherbutters

Cheryl's Berry-Berry Cocktail

Ingredients

1/2 Cup Coconut Water

1 Large Starfruit

1 Heaping Tbsp Moringa Powder

1 Cup Kale

1/2 Cup Woon Choy or Pakchoy

1/2 Cup Watercress

1 Custard Apple or Naseberry

1 Banana

1 Small piece of St. Andrew Black Mint

Method

Add the Starfruit to the Coconut Water and blend until liquefied.

Add the Woon Choy and blend until smooth.

Do the final blending with the Banana and Custard Apple and Black Mint Leaves.

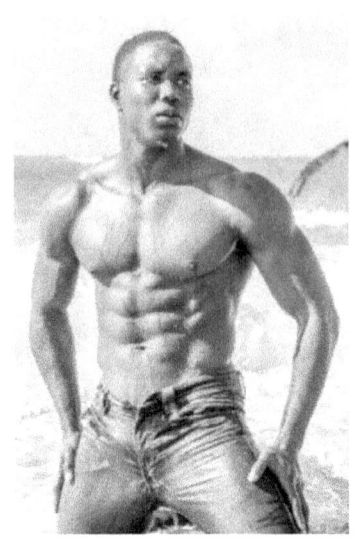

Clifton "Zeus" Lee

Fitness Model & Personal Trainer

Clifton's Glowing Green Smoothie

I have this almost every morning and I can truly say that it has made me feel and look my best in a short period of time.

Ingredients

2 1/2 Cups Cold Water

6 Cups Spinach, chopped

8 Cups Romaine Lettuce, chopped

2 Cups Celery, chopped

1 Cup Pineapple, diced

2 Tbsp. Lime Juice

Method

Add Water and chopped Greens to the blender.

Start the blender on a low speed, blend until smooth.

Increase the speed and add the Pineapple and the Lime Juice.

Makes 60oz.

Substitution

3 Tbsp. Lemon Juice may be used instead of the Lime Juice

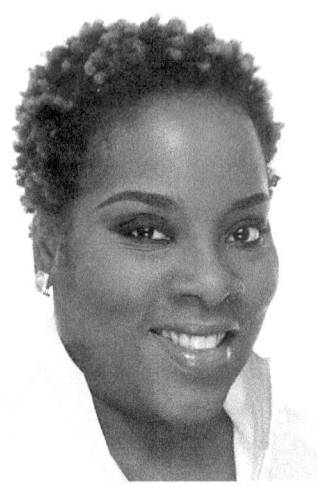

Dayna
Wallace

Online
Marketing
Specialist

Dayna's Morning Fuel

This is my breakfast smoothie and it's DELISH! Eating healthy doesn't have to taste bad.

Ingredients

2 Handfuls of Shredded Callaloo Leaves

1 Cup Soy Milk

1 Cup Irish Moss

3 Cups Pawpaw (plus 1/2 the Seeds)

1 Tbsp Flax Seeds, Ground

Method

Blend the Callaloo in the Soy Milk until liquefied.

Add the Irish Moss, Pawpaw, Pawpaw Seeds and Flax Seeds to the blender jar.

Blend until smooth.

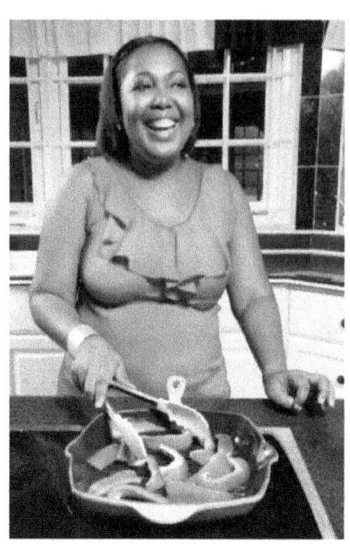

Jacqui
"The Juicy Chef"
Sinclair

Food Stylist
& Director of
Kingston Kitchen

Juicy Chef's Callaloo Colada

One day I was craving a Piña Colada, and made this delicious green smoothie. It has become a staple for me whenever I crave a natural sweet treat.

Ingredients

2 Cups Callaloo Leaves (Tightly Packed)

3/4 Cup Moringa Leaves

2 Honey Bananas, cut into chunks

1 Cup East Indian Mango, cut into chunks

1 Cup Sugarloaf Pineapple, cut into chunks

2 Cups Cold Unsweetened Coconut Milk

1 Tbsp Ground Organic Flaxseeds

Method

Add all of the above ingredients and blend until smooth and creamy.

Pour into 2 large glasses and serve immediately.

Serves 2

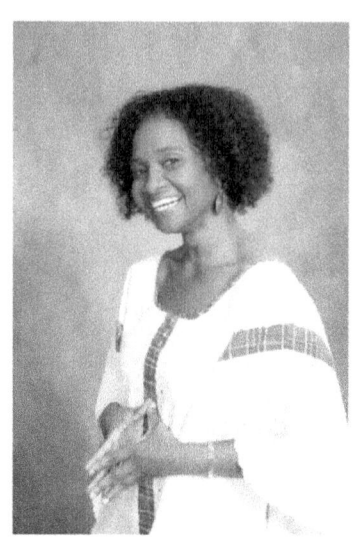

Jo-Ann
Richards

Author &
Ethnomusicologist

Jo-Ann's Power Up

The truth is, until Didan came along with the Jamaican Green Smoothie Challenge, my mom and I just threw stuff in, blended and we drank it! Sometimes it tasted great. Sometimes, it was just drinkable. But, this is one of my favourite blends, so I hope you like it.

Ingredients

1 Cup Callaloo Leaves

1 Cup Pak Choy, Parsley & Moringa

1 Cup Coconut Water

2 Frozen Bananas

1/2 Cup Frozen Soursop

1 Small Pawpaw

Method

Blend the Greens in Coconut Water until all the bits have been liquefied.

Add the fruits and then blend it until everything is smooth.

Serves 1

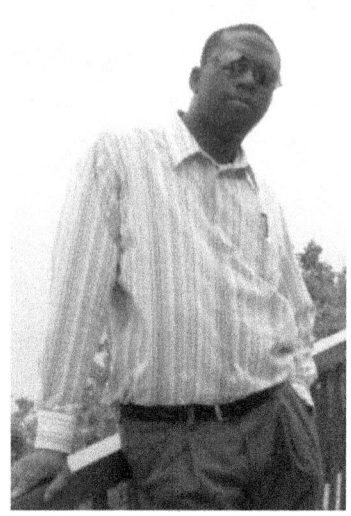

Kamaaleo
Burnett

Minister of
Religion

Kamaaleo's Green Vibrance

Ingredients

1 Cup Callaloo Leaves, chopped

1 Cup Lettuce, shredded

1-2 Cups Almond Milk

1 Banana, sliced 1 Apple, cored and chopped 2 Prunes

Method

Blend Callaloo and Lettuce in the Almond Milk until liquefied.

Add the Banana, Apple and Prunes, then blend until smooth.

Serves 1.

Substitution

You may use Coconut Water instead of Almond Milk.

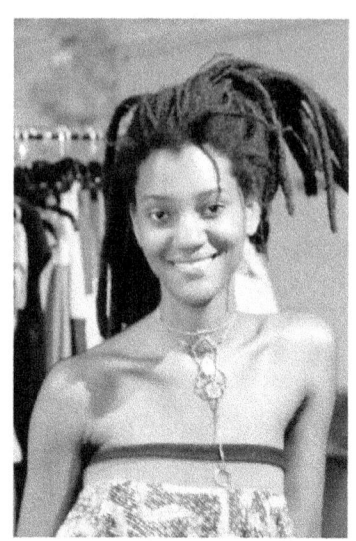

Mamayashi

Fashion
Designer

Mamayashi's Green Dream

Ingredients

2 Otaheite Apples

1 1/2 Cups Watermelon

1 Handful Sweet Basil

Method

Remove the seeds from the Apples and chop them up.

Remove the seeds and rind from the Watermelon and chop up the flesh.

Add the fruit and Basil leaves to the blender jar and blended all the ingredients until smooth.

Serves 3.

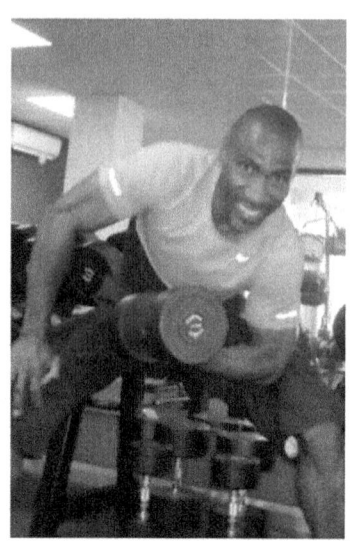

Michael
McKenzie

Certified
Personal
Trainer

Michael's Green Power for Men

Ingredients

1/2 Cup Callaloo

1/2 Cup Spinach

1 Cup Coconut Water

1/2 Large Cucumber

1/2 Cup Pumpkin Seeds

1 Large Banana

1/2 Large Avocado

1 Tbsp Moringa Powder

Method

Blend Callaloo and Spinach in Coconut Water until liquefied.

Add Cucumber and Pumpkin Seeds then blend until liquefied.

Add Banana, Avocado and Moringa Powder and blend until smooth.

Substitutions

You may use 2 tbsp Cherbutters Pumpkin Seed Butter in place of the Pumpkin Seeds.

Monique
"Irie Diva"
Solomon

Lifestyle
Blogger

Irie Diva's Weight Loss Thickie

My Magic Bullet Blender makes it very easy to blend my green smoothie and take it with me.

Ingredients

1 Handful Mixed Lettuce

1 Handful Spinach

1 Handful Kale

1 Cup freshly, squeezed Orange Juice

2 Tbsp Flax Seeds

1 Banana, frozen

1 Handful Blueberries

Method

Pack the blender cup with the ingredients, in the order listed, then screw on the cap.

Pulse the blender until the ingredients are chopped up. Then twist and let it blend until smooth.

Substitutions

If you can't find Blueberries, you may use East Indian Mangoes instead.

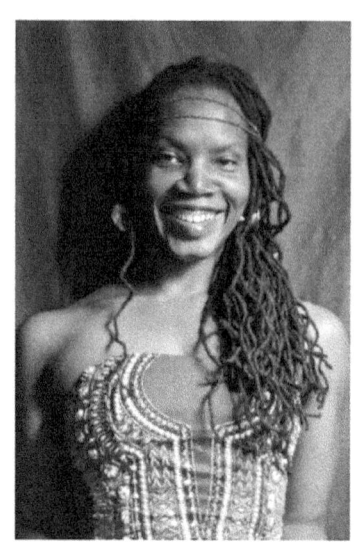

Sabriya
Simon

Photographer

Sabriya's Coco-Cocoa Bowl

Ingredients

2 Cups Kale

1 Sprig Mint Leaves

1 Cup Coconut Water

2 Cups Mango, chunks

1 Cup Banana, chunks

1 Tsp Pomegranate Powder

1/2 Tsp Cinnamon (ground)

1 Lime, juiced

1 Tbsp Cacao Nibs

1 Tbsp Shredded Coconut

Method

Blend the Kale and Mint leaves in the Coconut Water until liquefied.

Add the rest of ingredients, then blend until smooth. Serve in your favourite bowl.

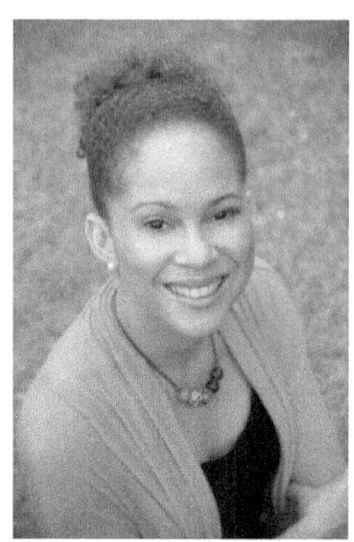

Stacey Aiken

Lifestyle &
Health Coach

Stacey's Zip-Zap

Ingredients

3 oz or 1/2 a Medium Cucumber, de-seeded

4 oz or 3 Pineapple Slices, core removed

3oz or 1 Medium Ripe Banana

1 oz or a Generous Handful of Tender Callaloo Leaves

1 Tsp Moringa (Powdered)

1/2 oz Cilantro Leaves

4-6 oz Coconut Water

Method

Place ingredients in blender and blend until smooth

Makes 10-12oz.

Substitutions

You may use freshly, squeezed Orange Juice instead of the Coconut Water.

References

Ann Wigmore Natural Health Institute, Inc.,
http://www.annwigmore.org/living_foods.html.

The Green Smoothie Community.
http://greensmoothiecommunity.com/2012/02/20/to-juice-or-bl
end-2/.

Green Smoothie Revolution.
http://greensmoothiesblog.com/blending-vs-juicing/.

"Jamaica Faces Non-Communicable Disease Epidemic -
Ferguson." *The Jamaica Gleaner*, March 13, 2014. Accessed 5 May
2014.
http://jamaica-gleaner.com/gleaner/20140313/news/news3.html.

Wigmore, Ann. *Rebuild Your Health: With High Energy
Enzyme Nourishment.* New Mexico: Ann Wigmore Foundation,
1991.

About the Author

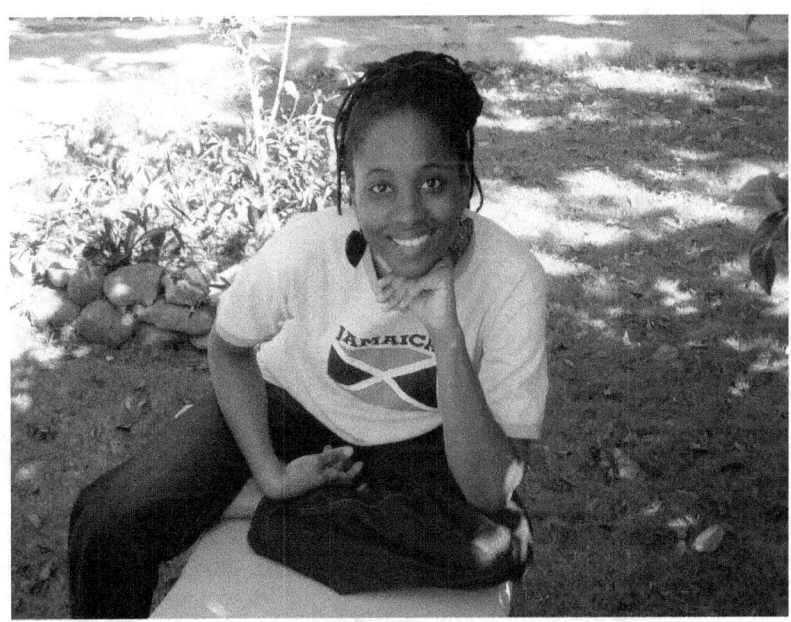

    Didan Ashanta is a natural living enthusiast who blogs about gentle parenting, whole-food plant-based eats and her cross-cultural exploits at <u>DidanAshanta.com</u>. A Jamaican expat living in Japan, she works as a Freelance Writer and English Teacher, and enjoys developing hearty and healthy recipes under the 'Eat Jamaican' theme. Didan combines her training, as an Educator and Counsellor (LifeStylist), with her years of experience, in the food service industry, to encourage healthy living through tasty dining. The heart and brain behind the Jamaican Green Smoothie movement, she believes and continues to prove that lives can be transformed, one cup at a time.

Grab Your FREE Gift!

Congrats on taking the first step towards improving your health and wellness!

Just for downloading "Jamaican Green Smoothies", I'm giving you access to the wildly popular 30-Day Jamaican Green Smoothie Challenge eGuide! Type this link into your browser to get started: http://bit.ly/FREEJGSGift

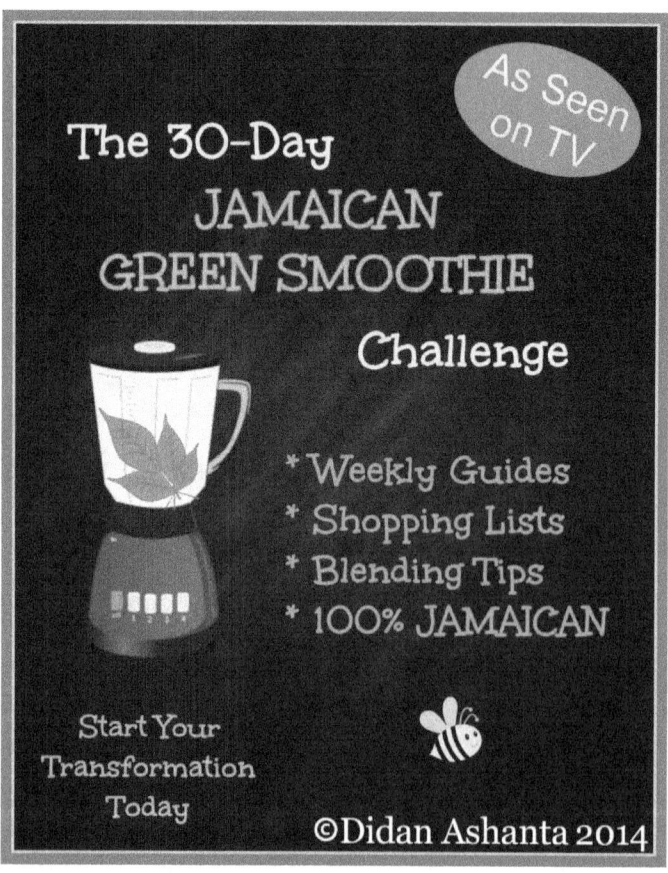